Metabolic Mastery:

Ditch Your Diet, Shed Fat, and

Maintain a Healthy Lifestyle

By

Dr. Laura J. Crawford

Copyright © by Dr. Laura J. Crawford 2024.

All rights reserved.

Table of Content

Introduction

Once upon a time, a group of friends wanted to lose weight and live a better lifestyle, like many of us. They tried every diet imaginable, from low-carb to low-fat, juice cleanses to fasting, but no matter how hard they tried, the outcomes were always the same: brief success followed by eventual disappointment.

Frustrated and frustrated, they began to wonder if they were missing anything—something other than fad diets and current training routines. That's when they discovered the secret to long-term weight loss and good health: Metabolic Mastery.

But before we get into their journey and the transformational impact of metabolic mastery, let's define metabolism and why it's the key to realizing your body's full potential.

Understanding Metabolism.

Imagine your body as a highly tuned mechanism that is continuously working to keep you alive and performing well. Your metabolism, which transforms food and drink into energy, is at the core of this machine. It's what keeps your heart pumping, your lungs breathing, and your cells growing and healing.

What is Metabolism?

Metabolism is commonly thought of as the pace at which your body burns calories, but it is much more than that. To sustain life, your cells undergo a complicated sequence of chemical interactions. There are two main parts of your metabolism:

- Basal Metabolic Rate (BMR): The number of calories required for basic functions like breathing, blood circulation, and cell repair at rest.

- Total Daily Energy Expenditure (TDEE): The total number of calories burned in a day, including BMR and physical activity.

How Metabolism Impacts Weight Loss

Now, this is where things become interesting. Your metabolism determines whether you lose, gain, or retain your present weight. When you consume more calories than your body requires, the extra energy is stored as fat for later use. On the other side, when you consume fewer calories than your body requires, it burns stored fat for energy, causing weight loss.

But here is the kicker: not all calories are created equal, and not all weight loss solutions are sustainable. Crash diets and excessive calorie restriction may result in quick weight reduction at first, but they can also hurt your metabolism, slowing it down and making future weight loss more difficult.

Common Metabolism Myths Busted

Before we go, let's refute some common metabolic fallacies that may be preventing you from accomplishing your health and fitness goals:

- Myth #1: Metabolism is completely regulated by genetics. While genetics influence your metabolic rate, a variety of lifestyle factors, such as nutrition, exercise, sleep, and stress levels, can also have an impact.

- Myth #2: Eating small, frequent meals increases your metabolism. While eating regular meals will help keep your metabolism running smoothly, the amount and substance of those meals are just as important as the frequency.

- Myth #3: Certain meals can boost your metabolism. While certain meals may have a mild thermogenic impact, which means they temporarily enhance your metabolic rate, there is no silver bullet for boosting your metabolism.

- Myth #4: Metabolism slows down with age. While it is true that your metabolism slows as you get older, this is not an unavoidable component of aging. Maintaining a healthy lifestyle may help you keep your metabolism running smoothly into your golden years.

Now that we've cleared up some common myths regarding metabolism, let's delve deeper into the field of metabolic mastery and learn how to discard your diet, lose weight, and live a healthy lifestyle for good. So grab a cup of tea, sit down, and get ready to start on a trip that will change the way you think about food, exercise, and your body's great potential.

Chapter 1: Problems with Traditional Diets

Dieting was once the most popular notion in a culture preoccupied with fast remedies and rapid satisfaction. Everywhere you went, there were promises of quick weight loss, slimming smoothies, and miraculous medications that claimed to burn fat overnight. However, for many others, including myself, dieting was everything from miraculous. Instead of attaining their long-term weight reduction and robust health goals, many became locked in a cycle of yo-yo dieting, frustration, and despair.

The Yo-Yo Dieting Cycle.

I have been on diets for as long as I can remember, Whether it was the newest celebrity-endorsed fad diet or a well-intentioned attempt to eat healthier, I was constantly on the lookout for the next fast cure that would finally help me shed those pesky pounds. And for a time, I thought I'd found the answer. The pounds would melt away, my clothing would fit better, and I would feel like I had regained control of my body and life.

But eventually, the weight would creep back on. Perhaps a stressful incident or a holiday season full of enticing snacks and lavish meals drove me off course. Whatever the cause, the outcome was always the same: I was back where I started, or worse off than before. So the cycle would start again: another diet, another round of fleeting success, and another unavoidable failure.

It wasn't until I stepped back and saw the larger picture that I understood how harmful this yo-yo dieting cycle was. Not only was it wreaking havoc on my self-esteem and emotional health, but it was also hurting my physique and metabolism.

Why Long-Term Diets Don't Work

The fact is that diets do not work. Sure, you may have some initial success, but more often than not, the weight you lose returns with a fury as soon as you stop the diet. Why? Because most diets are unsustainable in the long run. They focus on rigorous calorie restriction, excluding whole food categories, or eliminating your favorite meals. And, while these tactics may help you lose weight quickly, they are unrealistic and unsustainable in the long run.

Diets are unsuccessful for more reasons than merely their lack of durability. A psychological component is also included. When you start on a diet, you are effectively telling yourself that you cannot eat particular things, which makes you desire them even more. This might cause feelings of deprivation, guilt, and humiliation, which can eventually undermine your weight loss attempts.

Then there's the physiological component. When you severely limit your calorie intake, your body enters famine mode, lowering your metabolism and storing fat for survival. This can make it much more difficult to shed weight and keep it off in the long run.

Metabolic Damage: The Hidden Cost of Dieting

But the most insidious side effect of yo-yo dieting is the harm it does to your metabolism. Your metabolism functions like a fragile ecosystem, perfectly adjusted to keep your body working smoothly and effectively. However, subjecting it to the ups and downs of yo-yo dieting disrupts this delicate equilibrium.

When you severely reduce your caloric intake, your body responds by lowering your metabolism to preserve energy. This implies that when you eventually stop dieting and resume eating regularly, your metabolism slows, making it simpler to gain weight and more difficult to lose it.

However, a slowdown in your metabolism is not the only cause for concern. Yo-yo dieting can also lead to insulin resistance, a condition in which your cells become less receptive to insulin, the hormone that regulates blood sugar levels. This can raise your chance of developing type 2 diabetes, heart disease, and other major health issues.

Yo-yo dieting can also disrupt your hunger hormones, leaving you continuously hungry and boosting your desire for high-calorie, high-fat meals. This can lead to a vicious cycle of overeating and weight gain, escalating the problem.

In summary, yo-yo dieting results in a lose-lose situation. It not only fails to provide long-term weight reduction outcomes, but it can also harm your metabolism and health. So, if diets don't work, what are the alternatives? How can you accomplish long-term weight loss and vigorous health without falling into the trap of yo-yo dieting? That is what we will investigate in the following pages. So take a cup of tea, relax, and prepare to experience the transformational power of metabolic mastery.

Chapter 2: Metabolic Solution

Traditional diets frequently fail to deliver long-term weight loss and healthy health, leaving us feeling disappointed, starved, and discouraged. What if there was another way? What if we switched our attention from restricted diets and calorie tracking to something more fundamental: our metabolism? Welcome to Chapter 2 of "Metabolic Mastery: Ditch Your Diet, Shed Fat, and Maintain a Healthy Lifestyle," where we'll look at the metabolic answer to long-term weight loss and good health.

Eating for Metabolic Health.

Regarding reaching and maintaining a healthy weight, what you eat is just as important as how much you consume. Instead of focusing on calorie tracking and portion management, the key to metabolic mastery is eating the proper meals that support your metabolism and general health.

So, what does it mean to eat for metabolic health? It's all about fueling your body with nutrient-dense, complete foods that include the critical vitamins, minerals, and antioxidants it requires to flourish. This entails focusing on meals that are high in:

- **Protein**: Protein is necessary for tissue formation and repair, muscular development, and hormone regulation. Incorporate a source of lean protein into each meal, such as chicken, fish, tofu, beans, or Greek yogurt.

- **Healthy Fats:** Unlike common opinion, not all fats are unhealthy for you. In reality, healthy fats are a vital component of a well-balanced diet since they assist brain function, hormone synthesis, and nutrition absorption. Include healthy fat sources in your meals daily, such as avocados, almonds, seeds, olive oil, and fatty seafood like salmon.

- **Complex Carbohydrates**: Carbohydrates have a poor name, but they're a crucial source of energy for your body and brain. The idea is to select complex carbs rich in fiber and minerals yet low in refined sugars and processed substances. Consider whole grains such as quinoa, brown rice, oats, fruits, vegetables, and legumes.

- **Fruits and Vegetables**: Provide vitamins, minerals, and antioxidants that promote overall health and metabolism. Fill half of your plate with colorful fruits and veggies at each meal to ensure you obtain a diverse range of nutrients.

By concentrating on nutrient-dense, whole foods and paying attention to the quality of your diet rather than the quantity, you can nourish your body from the inside out and promote optimal metabolic health.

Understanding Macronutrients

In addition to selecting the proper meals, knowing the role of macronutrients in your diet is critical for optimizing your metabolism and attaining long-term weight reduction. Macronutrients, or macros for short, are the three primary energy-producing components of food: protein, carbs, and fat.

- **Protein**: Protein is commonly referred to as the "building block of life," and with good reason. It is necessary for tissue growth and repair, muscle development, and hormone regulation. In addition to its involvement in metabolism, protein helps you feel full and satisfied, making it an essential component of any weight-reduction diet.

- **Carbohydrates**: Carbohydrates are your body's primary source of energy, fueling your muscles and brain. While carbohydrates have received a negative reputation in recent years, not all carbs are created equal. Complex carbs, such as those found in whole grains, fruits, and vegetables, are high in fiber and minerals, which can help to regulate blood sugar levels and promote general health.

- **Fats**: Healthy fats are an important element of a well-balanced diet since they promote brain function, hormone synthesis, and nutrient absorption. While fats contain more calories than protein and carbs, they are essential for regulating metabolism and encouraging satiety. Avocados, almonds, seeds, and olive oil are good sources of healthy fats to include in your daily diet.

Understanding the significance of macronutrients in your diet and ensuring you obtain the proper balance of protein, carbs, and fats will help you feed your body effectively, promote optimal metabolic function, and achieve long-term weight loss and good health.

Hormones and Metabolism

The truth about metabolism is much more complex than the simple "calories in, calories out" equation that many people believe. Your metabolism is controlled by a complex network of hormones, neurotransmitters, and other biochemical messengers that dictate when your body should burn fat, store energy, or build muscle.

One of the primary hormones involved in metabolism is insulin. Your pancreas secretes insulin in reaction to elevated blood sugar levels, which facilitates the transfer of glucose from the circulation into your cells for use as an energy source. Your blood sugar levels rise after eating a meal high in carbs, and your pancreas releases insulin to lower them. On the other hand, persistently high insulin levels can cause insulin resistance, a state in which your cells lose their sensitivity to insulin's effects. This condition raises your blood sugar levels and increases your chance of developing type 2 diabetes and other metabolic diseases.

Leptin is another significant hormone that affects metabolism. Your fat cells generate the hormone leptin, which signals your brain to control appetite and energy expenditure. When fat stores are sufficient, leptin levels increase, telling your brain to stop eating when you're satisfied. Leptin resistance, on the other hand, can affect overweight or obese people. In this case, the brain becomes less susceptible to leptin's effects, which increase appetite and overeating.

Growth hormones, thyroid hormones, cortisol, and adrenaline are other hormones that affect metabolism and control hunger, energy expenditure, and fat storage. You may support ideal hormone balance and encourage a healthy metabolism by being aware of the function that hormones play in metabolism and how nutrition, lifestyle, and other variables might affect them. This entails maintaining stress levels, exercising often, eating a well-balanced diet full of foods high in nutrients, and placing a high value on rest and sleep.

 In conclusion, eating for metabolic health, comprehending the importance of macronutrients in your diet, and promoting optimum hormone balance are all parts of the metabolic answer to long-term weight loss and good health. You don't have to fall victim to yo-yo dieting and restrictive diets to achieve long-lasting weight reduction and robust health. Instead, you may promote healthy hormone balance, balance your consumption of protein, carbs, and fats, and feed your body with nutrient-dense, whole foods. Therefore, give up on the diet mindset, embrace metabolic mastery, and take permanent control of your health and well-being.

Chapter 3: Metabolic Mastery Approach

We will delve deeply into the concepts of metabolic mastery, examining how to create a balanced plate and the significance of meal timing in maximizing your metabolism and achieving long-lasting weight loss and vibrant health.

The Fundamentals of Metabolic Mastery

Fundamentally, metabolic mastery entails adopting a holistic perspective on health and wellness, emphasizing the development of nutrient-dense diets, appropriate metabolic support, and wholesome lifestyle practices that enhance general well-being. The following are some essential metabolic mastery concepts:

- **Emphasize Whole, Nutrient-Dense Foods:** Make a point of consuming whole, nutrient-dense foods that are a good source of vitamins, minerals, and antioxidants rather than depending on packaged, processed meals that are high in sugar, unhealthy fats, and empty calories. Fruits, vegetables, whole grains, lean meats, nuts, seeds, and healthy fats are all included in this.

- **Balance Your Macronutrients**: To support healthy metabolic function and promote satiety, try to incorporate a balance of protein, carbs, and fats in each meal. Protein aids in tissue growth and repair; healthy fats promote hormone synthesis and the body's ability to absorb nutrients; and carbs provide your muscles and brain energy.

- **Eat Mindfully**: Avoid distractions when eating and pay attention to your body's signals of hunger and fullness. This can encourage a positive relationship with food and help avoid overindulging.

- **Remain Hydrated:** To maintain optimal metabolic function and to keep hydrated, sip copious amounts of water throughout the day. Your metabolism will slow down if you're dehydrated, which will make you tired and perform poorly.

- **Prioritize Sleep and Stress Management**: To support optimum hormone balance and enhance general well-being, get enough sleep each night and engage in stress-reduction practices like yoga, deep breathing, and meditation.

- **Stay Active**: Include regular exercise in your daily regimen to preserve muscle mass, support metabolic health, and advance general fitness. For optimal effects, try a combination of aerobic, strength, and flexibility workouts.

You may promote proper metabolic function, nourish your body from the inside out, lose weight sustainably, and maintain robust health by adhering to these metabolic mastery principles.

Creating a Harmonious Plate

Building a balanced plate at every meal to ensure you're getting a wide variety of nutrients while supporting optimal metabolic function is one of the fundamentals of metabolic mastery. So what constitutes a balanced dish? This is an explanation:

- **Protein:** To begin, arrange a source of lean protein, such as beans, Greek yogurt, fish, chicken, or tofu, across a fourth of your plate. Protein is necessary for hormone regulation, tissue development and repair, and muscular growth.

- **Vegetables**: To receive important vitamins, minerals, and antioxidants, put half of your plate on colorful veggies. To make sure you're receiving a wide spectrum of nutrients, aim for a variety of colors and varieties, such as leafy greens, peppers, carrots, broccoli, and tomatoes.

- **Carbs**: Use a portion of complex carbs, such as quinoa, brown rice, sweet potatoes, or whole grains, to occupy the remaining quarter of your plate. Rich in minerals and fiber, complex carbs can help control blood sugar levels and encourage feelings of pleasure and fullness.

- **Healthy Fats**: To enhance hormone synthesis, nutritional absorption, and general health, add a portion of healthy fats to your meal in addition to avocado, nuts, seeds, or olive oil. To control calories, aim for a tiny piece that is around the size of your thumb.

You can make sure you're getting a wide range of nutrients to support normal metabolic function, encourage feelings of fullness and pleasure, lose weight sustainably, and maintain vigorous health by assembling a balanced plate at each meal.

The Importance of Timing Your Meals

The timing of your meals may affect not only how well your plate is balanced, but also how well your metabolism works and how well you reach your fitness and health objectives. Here are some important things to think about:

- **Consume Regularly**: To maintain a healthy metabolism and avoid energy slumps, try to consume meals and snacks regularly throughout the day. Blood sugar levels can be stabilized, and overeating later in the day can be avoided by eating every three to four hours.

- **Don't Miss Breakfast**: In terms of metabolism, breakfast is by far the most significant meal of the day. Within an hour of waking up, you may boost your metabolism, fuel your day, and avoid overindulging in the afternoon by having a nutritious breakfast.

- **Include Protein with Every Meal**: Since protein digests more slowly than fats or carbs, having a source of protein with every meal might help you feel fuller and less prone to overindulge, which may help with weight loss.

- **Be Aware of Evening Eating**: Although it's essential to nourish your body throughout the day, avoid eating late at night since this might cause weight gain and disturb your sleep. To give your body enough time to digest before bed, try to finish eating at least two to three hours before going to bed.

- **Listen to Your Body**: In the end, the meal that best suits your unique requirements and preferences is the one that you should schedule. Eat when you're hungry and stop when you're full, paying attention to your body's signals of hunger and fullness.

By carefully scheduling and distributing your snacks and meals throughout the day, you can avoid overindulging, promote optimal metabolic function, lose weight sustainably, and maintain healthy health.

To maintain optimal metabolic function and achieve sustained weight loss and robust health, the metabolic mastery method entails adopting important concepts, including emphasizing whole, nutrient-dense meals, assembling a balanced plate at each meal, and being mindful of meal time. By may maintain healthy metabolic function, feed your body from the inside out, and reach your lifelong fitness and health objectives by incorporating these ideas into your daily practice.

Chapter 4: Foods to Increase Your Metabolism

This chapter will cover a wide range of foods that boost metabolism, including superfoods for metabolic health, delectable recipes, meal ideas for optimal metabolic function, and supplements to improve your metabolism and general well-being. Now put on your apron and get ready to fuel your body internally!

Superfoods for Optimal Metabolism

Because they are high in nutrients, superfoods are particularly good for your health and well-being. They are brimming with nutrients that support normal metabolic function, increase energy, and advance general health, including vitamins, minerals, antioxidants, and other helpful components. Superfoods that are very good for metabolic health include the following:

- **Berries**: Rich in fiber, vitamins, and antioxidants, berries include blueberries, strawberries, raspberries, and blackberries. They're the ideal complement to your diet to support metabolic health because they're high in taste and low in calories.

- **Leafy Greens**: Leafy greens like collard greens, Swiss chard, spinach, and kale are a powerhouse of nutrients. They include high levels of iron, calcium, and vitamins A, C, and K. Additionally, leafy greens are high in fiber, maintain a healthy digestive system, and aid in creating sensations of fullness.

- **Salmon**: Omega-3 fatty acids, which are abundant in fatty fish like salmon, mackerel, and sardines, have been demonstrated to promote heart health, lower inflammation, and increase metabolism. Additionally, omega-3 fatty acids may lower the likelihood of insulin resistance and help control insulin levels.

- **Avocado**: Packed with vitamins, fiber, and good fats, avocados are a great option for supporting metabolic health. Avocados include monounsaturated fats that can enhance feelings of fullness and aid in weight reduction. Additionally, the fiber in avocados helps to maintain good digestion and blood sugar levels.

- **Quinoa**: Packed with protein, fiber, and vital vitamins and minerals, quinoa is a whole grain free of gluten. Moreover, it is a complete protein, which means that it has all nine of the necessary amino acids required by your body for optimal activity. Quinoa is a great choice for encouraging feelings of fullness and maintaining a healthy metabolism.

- **Green Tea**: Studies have indicated that the antioxidants included in green tea, known as catechins, can increase metabolism and encourage fat burning. Regularly consuming green tea may boost energy expenditure and aid in weight reduction.

Including these superfoods regularly in your diet can support normal metabolic function, increase energy, and improve general health and well-being.

Meal Ideas and Recipes to Boost Metabolism

Now that you know about the foods that can increase your metabolism, let's put them into practice with some delectable meal ideas and dishes that will satisfy your hunger and give you a surge of energy. We have everything you need, whether you're searching for a quick and simple breakfast, a filling lunch, or a nutritious dinner.

- **Breakfast**: A smoothie consisting of Greek yogurt, almond milk, and a handful of mixed berries may be a great way to start the day since it speeds up metabolism. Alternatively, try a large dish of overnight oats garnished with chopped almonds, sliced bananas, and honey.

- **Lunch**: Prepare a salmon salad with mixed greens, avocado, cherry tomatoes, and a squeeze of lemon and olive oil for a filling midday meal. An additional option for a high-protein lunch that will leave you feeling full and energized all afternoon is quinoa and veggies stir-fried with chicken or tofu.

- Dinner: How about grilled salmon fillet with steamed broccoli and roasted sweet potatoes for dinner? Make a pot of turkey and black bean chili, rich with seasonings and vegetables, for a filling and healthy dinner that's ideal for cold nights.

- **Snacks**: Consume metabolism-boosting snacks such as hummus-topped carrot sticks, Greek yogurt with berries and granola, or a handful of mixed nuts and seeds to maintain your energy levels in between meals.

You can fuel your body with nutrient-rich meals that support optimal metabolic function, encourage long-lasting weight reduction, and promote robust health by incorporating these metabolism-boosting recipes and meal ideas into your daily routine.

Supplements that Help You Burn Fat

To support your metabolism and general well-being, you may also think about taking supplements in addition to eating meals that increase energy levels. Supplements can assist you when needed, but they should never replace a balanced diet and way of life. The following nutrients might aid in maintaining metabolic health:

- **Omega-3 Fatty Acids**: Known for their anti-inflammatory qualities, omega-3 fatty acids, which are present in fish oil supplements, may improve heart health, lower inflammation, and encourage a healthy metabolism.

- **Probiotics**: Supplements with probiotics include good microorganisms that promote gut health and a healthy digestive system. For general health and maybe to promote metabolic function, gut flora equilibrium must be maintained.

- **Vitamin D**: An essential component of several metabolic processes, insulin sensitivity, energy synthesis, and immunological function are all dependent on vitamin D. Vitamin D deficiency is common, especially in the winter when there is less sun exposure; thus, for certain people, taking supplements of vitamin D may be helpful.

- **Green Tea Extract**: Catechins, the antioxidants in green tea, are believed to increase metabolism and encourage fat burning. Green tea extract is a concentrated concentration of these antioxidants. Using a green tea extract supplement might promote a healthy metabolism and weight loss.

- **Caffeine**: A natural stimulant, caffeine can raise energy levels and speed up the metabolism. Although there are supplements containing caffeine, it's crucial to take them sparingly and be aware of how they affect your body.

It's crucial to speak with a healthcare provider before incorporating any supplements into your regimen to be sure they're safe and suitable for you, particularly if you take medication or have any underlying medical concerns.

In conclusion, you may support healthy metabolic function, increase energy levels, and encourage long-lasting weight reduction and robust health by including foods, recipes, and supplements that stimulate metabolism in your daily routine. Through nutrient-dense meals, regular exercise, and a strong emphasis on self-care, you may attain metabolic mastery and then assume lifelong responsibility for your health and overall well-being.

Chapter 5: Lifestyle Strategies for a Healthy Metabolism

We'll be discussing the vital impact that lifestyle variables play in maintaining a healthy metabolism in this chapter of "Metabolic Mastery: Ditch Your Diet, Shed Fat, and Maintain a Healthy Lifestyle." We'll go over the key strategies—exercise, stress reduction, and sleep, among others—that you can employ to optimize your metabolic health, achieve sustainable weight loss, and preserve good health.

Exercise's Significance for Metabolic Health

Regular exercise is essential for increasing metabolism and promoting general health and well-being. Exercise has a significant influence on metabolic health in addition to burning calories and assisting you in maintaining a healthy weight. How to do it is as follows:

- **Increases Muscle Mass**: Building more muscle is one of the best methods to speed up your metabolism. Muscle tissue burns more calories at rest than fat tissue does because of its higher metabolic activity. You may develop and maintain lean muscle mass by doing resistance training activities like weightlifting, bodyweight exercises, or resistance band workouts.

This will support your weight reduction efforts by raising your basal metabolic rate.

- **Improves Insulin Sensitivity****: Physical activity increases insulin sensitivity, which makes it easier for your cells to absorb glucose from the blood and utilise it as fuel. In addition to lowering the risk of insulin resistance, type 2 diabetes, and other metabolic problems, this can help control blood sugar levels.

- **Boosts Metabolic Rate**: Physical activity raises your body's resting metabolic rate, or the amount of calories burned. Exercises that are high in intensity, like circuit training or interval training, can momentarily increase your metabolic rate even more, resulting in increased calorie burning and fat loss.

- **Promotes Fat Reduction**: Exercise has a long-lasting effect on fat reduction but it also burns calories during the act. Frequent exercise can aid in the reduction of visceral fat, which is the kind of fat deposited deep inside the belly and linked to a higher risk of metabolic syndrome, heart disease, and other health issues. This is especially true when exercise is accompanied by a nutritious diet.

Aim for two or more days of strength training in addition to at least 150 minutes of moderate-intensity aerobic activity or 75 minutes of vigorous-intensity aerobic activity every week, such activities that target all major muscle groups, to maximize the metabolic advantages of exercise. To get the most out of your workout and keep your body guessing, change up your cardio, weight training, and flexibility activities.

Techniques for Stress Management

For many people in today's fast-paced world, stress has become a way of life. Even while some stress is acceptable and even required for life, prolonged stress can negatively impact your overall health and metabolism. Here are some tips for successfully managing stress and how it impacts metabolism:

- **Impacts Hormone Levels**: Prolonged stress can throw the body's hormonal equilibrium off balance, which raises cortisol levels—the main stress hormone. Increased hunger, desires for high-calorie meals, and the development of belly fat are all consequences of elevated cortisol levels, which can impair metabolism and cause weight gain.

- **Promotes Emotional Eating**: Emotional eating and bad food choices are often the result of people using food as a coping technique when they're under stress. Stress eating can cause hormones related to appetite to be disturbed, leading to an increase in the desire for high-calorie, high-fat meals, overeating, and weight gain.

- **Disturbs Sleep**: Stress can affect the length and quality of sleep, which can result in weariness, agitation, and slowed metabolism. Sleep deprivation alters hunger hormones, increases appetite, and lowers energy expenditure, which makes it more difficult to have a healthy metabolism and lose weight.

Work stress management practices into your daily routine to maintain a healthy metabolism and efficiently manage stress. This might involve actions like:

- **Mindfulness Meditation**: This technique can foster relaxation, lower stress levels, and enhance general well-being. Every day, set aside a little period to sit still, concentrate on your breathing, and develop a sense of presence and serenity.
- **Yoga**: Yoga enhances flexibility and strength while promoting relaxation and lowering stress levels via a combination of physical postures, breathing techniques, and meditation. Include a daily yoga

practice in your regimen to enhance metabolic health and assist with stress management.

- **Deep Breathing Exercises**: Progressive muscle relaxation and diaphragmatic breathing are two examples of deep breathing techniques that can assist trigger the body's relaxation response, lower stress levels, and foster feelings of peace and well-being.

- **Regular Exercise**: Exercise improves mental and emotional health in addition to physical health. Frequent exercise supports a healthy metabolism by lowering stress levels, elevating mood, and enhancing sleep quality.

You may lower your stress levels, maintain a healthy metabolism, and advance your general health and well-being by implementing these stress-reduction strategies into your daily routine.

Sleep: Its Significance for Metabolism

Sleep is vital for controlling hunger, energy expenditure, and hormone balance, yet it is frequently disregarded in the context of weight reduction and metabolic health. The following are some methods to enhance sleep quality and promote metabolic health, as well as how sleep influences metabolism:

- **Controls Hunger Hormones**: Lack of sleep can mess with the hormones that regulate hunger, causing ghrelin, which promotes hunger, to rise and leptin, which indicates fullness, to fall. Increased hunger, desires for meals high in calories, and overindulging can result from this, all of which can impair metabolism and cause weight gain.

- **Impacts on Energy consumption**: Sleep deprivation can lower energy consumption, making weight loss and calorie burning more difficult. Lack of sleep can also result in tiredness, a drop in physical activity, and poor performance during exercise, which lowers metabolic rate and calorie burn even more.

- **Impacts Insulin Sensitivity**: Sleep is essential for controlling insulin sensitivity and blood sugar levels. Lack of sleep can affect an individual's ability to use insulin, which can raise blood sugar levels, build insulin resistance, and increase the risk of type 2 diabetes and other metabolic diseases.

Try implementing the following techniques into your nighttime routine to enhance metabolic health and improve the quality of your sleep:

- **Create a Regular Sleep Schedule**: To control your body's internal clock and enhance the quality of your sleep, go to bed and wake up at the same time every day, including on the weekends.

- **Create a soothing Bedtime Routine**: To tell your body it's time to wind down and get ready for sleep, create a soothing bedtime routine. This might involve doing things like reading, having a warm bath, using relaxation methods, or enjoying peaceful music.
- **Create a Sleep-Friendly Environment****: Furnish your bedroom with a cozy, tranquil space that promotes restful sleep. To encourage sound sleep, keep the space cold, quiet, and dark. You should also have comfy cushions and a mattress.
- **Reduce Screen Exposure**: In the hour before going to bed, spend less time in front of screens, including computers, tablets, cellphones, and televisions. Screen blue light can interfere with melatonin synthesis and cause sleep patterns to be disturbed.
- **Reduce Stimulants**: Steer clear of alcohol, nicotine, and caffeine in the hours before bed since they can disturb sleep patterns and impair the quality of your sleep.

Prioritizing sleep and implementing these techniques into your nighttime routine can help you get better quality sleep, maintain metabolic health, and enhance your general well-being.

To sum up, a healthy metabolism, long-term weight loss, and vital health are all greatly influenced by lifestyle choices. You may attain your lifelong fitness and health objectives by optimizing your metabolic health via regular exercise, stress management practices, sleep prioritization, and other healthy lifestyle choices. Try out several tactics to see which one suits you the most, and always pay attention to your body's signals and put your health and well-being first. You can control your metabolism and reach your maximum potential for health and vitality by using lifestyle measures.

Chapter 6: Troubleshooting: Overcoming Plateaus and Setbacks

Greetings and welcome to Chapter 6 of "Metabolic Mastery: Ditch Your Diet, Shed Fat, and Maintain a Healthy Lifestyle." In this chapter, we'll examine tactics for overcoming setbacks and plateaus as well as discuss frequent issues that emerge on the path to metabolic mastery. We'll provide you with the skills and strategies you need to overcome obstacles and achieve long-term success, from weight loss plateaus to addressing metabolic resistance to preserving metabolic health for life.

Overcoming a Weight Loss Plateau

On the path to greater health, weight loss plateaus are frequent and can be difficult to overcome. Even with the best of intentions, you might discover that your weight reduction slows after weeks or months of improvement. Thankfully, there are some tactics you may use to overcome weight reduction plateaus and keep moving closer to your objectives:

- **Reevaluate Your Calorie Intake**: You may experience a plateau in your calorie requirements while you lose weight. To ensure that you're still in a calorie deficit to support weight loss, try reevaluating your calorie consumption and making the necessary adjustments.

- **Switch Up Your Workout Routine**: If you've been working out the same way for a long time, your body could have become accustomed to it, which could result in a plateau. To push your body in new ways, consider varying the length or intensity of your workouts, adding new activities, or trying out other kinds of exercise.

- **Surround Yourself with Strength Training**: Increasing your lean muscle mass through strength training will speed up your metabolism and encourage fat reduction. To encourage muscle growth and overcome plateaus, consider adding additional strength training activities to your regimen if you've been concentrating mostly on cardio.

- **Prioritize Stress Management and Sleep**: By upsetting hormone balance and escalating cravings for high-calorie meals, prolonged stress and sleep deprivation can both lead to weight loss plateaus. Make sure to prioritize deep breathing, yoga, meditation, and other stress-reduction methods in addition to obtaining enough sleep to promote metabolic health and overcome plateaus.

- **Remain Consistent:** To avoid giving up, it's critical to remember that plateaus are a natural part of the weight reduction process. Maintain consistency in your healthy routine, have faith in the process, and concentrate on the intangible benefits, such as heightened mood, greater energy, and an overall sense of well-being.

You may overcome weight loss plateaus and keep moving forward in the direction of your fitness and health objectives by putting these techniques into practice and exercising patience and persistence.

Handling resistance to metabolism

It is more difficult to lose weight and have a healthy metabolism when your body develops resistance to the effects of food and exercise, known as metabolic resistance. Numerous factors, like heredity, hormone imbalances, long-term stress, inadequate sleep, and a history of dieting, might contribute to this. The following are some methods for addressing metabolic resistance and getting beyond barriers to weight loss:

- **Address Underlying Health Issues**: It's critical to take care of any underlying medical conditions that could be causing or exacerbating your metabolic resistance. Speak with a medical expert to rule out any illnesses and create a customized strategy to suit your particular requirements.

- **Emphasize Quality, Not Quantity**: Rather than becoming fixated on calorie tracking and stringent diets, concentrate on providing your body with wholesome, nutrient-dense foods that promote metabolic health. To fuel your body and maintain optimal metabolic function, make eating a balanced diet full of fruits, vegetables, whole grains, lean proteins, and healthy fats a priority.

- **Include Interval Training**: Research has demonstrated the efficacy of high-intensity interval training (HIIT) in surmounting metabolic resistance and fostering lipolysis. Incorporate high-intensity interval training (HIIT) into your exercise regimen to push your body, increase your metabolism, and overcome fitness plateaus.

- **Practice Mindful Eating**: This entails eating mindfully, which means slowing down, savoring each mouthful, and being aware of your body's signals of hunger and fullness. Overeating may be avoided, stress can be decreased, and metabolic health can be supported by eating thoughtfully and paying attention to your body's cues.

- **Seek Support**: You don't have to handle metabolic resistance on your own. It can be difficult to manage. Seek assistance from loved ones, close friends, or a qualified coach who can offer support, accountability, and direction while you strive to overcome challenges and meet your fitness and health objectives.

You can overcome metabolic resistance and make progress toward long-term metabolic mastery by treating underlying health conditions, prioritizing quality over quantity, implementing interval training, engaging in mindful eating, and getting help.

Sustaining Lifelong Metabolic Health

Achieving metabolic mastery takes more than simply achieving a specific weight or body composition; it also requires forming wholesome lifestyle practices that promote lifelong optimal metabolic function. Here are some tips for achieving long-term success and maintaining metabolic health:

- **Sustainable Habits**: Put less emphasis on transient solutions or fad diets and more on creating long-lasting, sustainable habits. This entails maintaining an active lifestyle, eating balanced food, getting enough sleep, controlling stress, and placing a high value on self-care.

- **Remain Active**: Maintaining metabolic health and avoiding weight gain require regular physical activity. Make time for the activities you enjoy, such as yoga, cycling, swimming, dancing, or walking, and incorporate them into your daily routine.

- **Eat Mindfully**: Slow down, enjoy every meal, and pay attention to your body's signals of hunger and fullness as you eat. When eating, stay away from computers and multitasking, and concentrate on savoring your meal and the dining experience.

- **Prioritize Sleep**: To maintain metabolic health, control hunger hormones, and enhance general well-being, aim for 7-9 hours of good sleep every night. To improve the quality of your sleep, develop a peaceful nighttime habit, a regular sleep schedule, and a sleep-friendly environment.

- **Manage Stress**: It's critical to develop good coping mechanisms and relaxation techniques since long-term stress can negatively affect metabolic health. To lower stress and promote metabolic health, try stress-reduction methods like deep breathing, yoga, meditation, or time spent in nature.

- **Remain Adaptable**: Keep in mind that life is erratic and that it's acceptable to occasionally stray from your path. Aim for growth rather than perfection, and concentrate on making healthy decisions the majority of the time while allowing yourself room for flexibility and balance.

You may sustain metabolic health for life and have long-lasting success on your path to metabolic mastery by implementing these suggestions into your daily routine and being dedicated to your health and well-being.

In summary, breaking through plateaus and obstacles is an essential component of the metabolic mastery path; nevertheless, with the appropriate techniques and attitude, you may overcome obstacles and reach your fitness and health objectives. Never lose hope in your health and well-being—whether it's through overcoming weight loss plateaus, addressing metabolic resistance, or preserving metabolic health for the rest of your life. You may overcome challenges and achieve long-term success on your path to metabolic mastery if you are committed, resilient, and follow the guidelines presented in this chapter.

Chapter 7: Long-Term Achievement: Integrating Metabolic Mastery into Your Lifestyle

Best wishes! After starting your road to metabolic mastery, it's time to maintain your gains and create long-lasting lifestyle adjustments that will benefit your overall health and well-being. We'll look at how to make metabolic mastery a way of life in this chapter, including how to set up long-lasting routines, overcome obstacles, maintain motivation, and recognize and appreciate your accomplishments along the way.

Long-Term Viability of Health Habits

To achieve metabolic mastery, you must develop lifelong healthy behaviors rather than focusing only on achieving a particular weight or body composition. Focusing on sustainable lifestyle adjustments can help you reap long-term rewards and lay the groundwork for long-term success. You should think about implementing the following sustainable behaviors into your everyday routine:

- **Nourish Your Body with Whole Meals**: Make a point of feeding your body entire, nutrient-dense meals that are high in vitamins, minerals, and antioxidants rather than depending on crash diets or shortcuts. To promote good metabolic function and general health, load your plate with a mix of fruits, vegetables, lean proteins, whole grains, nuts, seeds, and healthy fats.

- **Remain Active Every Day**: Maintaining metabolic health, aiding in weight control, and fostering general well-being all depend on regular physical exercise. Make time for the things you like doing, like yoga, walking, cycling, swimming, or dancing, and incorporate them into your daily schedule. Aim for two or more days of strength training activities that work all of the major muscle groups, in addition to at least 150 minutes of moderate-intensity aerobic activity or 75 minutes a week of vigorously intense aerobic exercise.

- **Prioritize Sleep and Stress Management**: Two key elements of metabolic mastery are getting enough sleep and managing stress well. For the sake of your general well-being, appetite, hormone regulation, and metabolic health, try to get between seven and nine hours of good sleep every night. To lower stress and promote metabolic health, try stress-reduction methods like deep breathing, yoga, meditation, or time spent in nature.

- **Practice Mindful Eating**: This entails eating mindfully, which means slowing down, savoring each mouthful, and being aware of your body's signals of hunger and fullness. When eating, stay away from computers and multitasking, and concentrate on savoring your meal and the dining experience. Overeating may be avoided, stress can be decreased, and metabolic health can be supported by eating thoughtfully and paying attention to your body's cues.

- **Remain Hydrated**: To maintain optimal metabolic function and to keep hydrated, sip copious amounts of water throughout the day. Your metabolism will slow down if you're dehydrated, which will make you tired and perform poorly. Aim for eight to ten glasses of water a day, and modify your consumption according to your needs, the weather, and your degree of exercise.

By incorporating these sustainable behaviors into your daily routine, you can lay the groundwork for long-term success and reap the lifelong benefits of metabolic mastery.

Overcoming Obstacles and Maintaining Inspiration

Long-term success requires not just forming durable habits but also anticipating and overcoming obstacles that may appear along the way. To sustain metabolic mastery, one must remain tough and driven while overcoming obstacles, giving in to temptation, and managing hectic schedules. The following are some methods for conquering obstacles and maintaining motivation when traveling:

- **Set Realistic Goals**: Make reasonable expectations for yourself and divide your long-term objectives into smaller, more doable tasks. Along the way, acknowledge your accomplishments and try not to be too harsh on yourself if you run into difficulties or disappointments. Aim to implement small, long-lasting improvements that are consistent with your objectives and beliefs.

- **Find Your Why**: Get in touch with the inner drives and inspirations behind your desire to master metabolism. A strong sense of purpose may help you stay motivated and focused on your objectives even in the face of obstacles, whether they are related to health, energy, or setting a good example for those you care about.

- **Remain Adaptable**: Since life is unpredictable, it's acceptable to occasionally stray from your intended path. Instead of viewing setbacks as failures, view them as chances to improve and gain knowledge. To overcome obstacles and continue moving towards your goals, be adaptable and flexible, and be prepared to change course when necessary.

- **Seek Support**: Encircle yourself with friends, family, or others who share your values so they can support and inspire you along the way. Talk to people about your goals and challenges, and rely on them when you need help, direction, or responsibility.

- **Exercise Self-Compassion**: Show yourself kindness and compassion, particularly while facing challenges or hardships. Keep in mind that you are only human, and it's acceptable to make errors or not live up to your expectations. Give yourself the same consideration and compassion that you would a friend, and concentrate on making progress rather than perfection.

By implementing these tactics and maintaining your resolve and motivation, you can get beyond obstacles, get over setbacks, and continue on your path to long-term success with metabolic mastery.

Honoring Your Achievements and Persisting in Your Growth

As you make progress toward metabolic mastery, it's critical to recognize your accomplishments and your development. Celebrate your successes and give yourself credit for your hard work and devotion, whether it's hitting a personal best, reaching a milestone, or improving your health and well-being. Here are some ideas for acknowledging your accomplishments and carrying on:

- **Acknowledge Your Achievements***: Give yourself time to reflect on how far you've come and recognize the improvements you've made in your life. Honor your accomplishments, no matter how modest, and acknowledge the effort and commitment it took to get there.

- **Reward Yourself**: Celebrate your accomplishments and reinforce good conduct by treating yourself to a special treat or indulgence. Choose a reward that is significant to you and aligns with your objectives and values, whether it be a rejuvenating spa day, your favorite dish, or a new wardrobe.

- **Share Your Victories**: Congratulate yourself and your group on your accomplishments by sharing your victories. Sharing your path, whether with friends, family, or neighbors, may encourage and inspire others and reaffirm your dedication to ongoing development and achievement.

- **Create New Goals**: Keep pushing yourself to new limits and use your accomplishments as inspiration to create new objectives. To achieve your goals, push yourself to continue developing and growing, whether it's by enhancing your physical well-being, learning a new skill, or working on a passion project.

- **Practice Gratitude**: Set aside some time every day to develop an attitude of thankfulness for all of life's benefits and the strides you've made toward metabolic mastery. Pay attention to the good things in your life and the upcoming opportunities for growth and fulfillment.

You may sustain momentum and remain dedicated to your lifelong quest toward metabolic mastery by acknowledging and appreciating your accomplishments and going on with your growth.

To sum up, achieving metabolic mastery is not the only thing that goes into this lifestyle; it also involves forming long-lasting habits, overcoming obstacles, maintaining motivation, and acknowledging your accomplishments along the way.

You may establish a habit of regularly implementing these tactics and maintaining your dedication to your health and well-being.

Lay the groundwork for sustained performance and reap the long-term benefits of metabolic mastery. Keep in mind that your path is unique to you, and acknowledge and appreciate your achievements at each stage of the process. You can succeed and prosper on your path to metabolic mastery if you use perseverance, determination, and the concepts covered in this chapter.

Conclusion: Your Journey to Metabolic Mastery

When you have finished reading "Metabolic Mastery: Ditch Your Diet, Shed Fat, and Maintain a Healthy Lifestyle," stop and consider the adventure you have already been on. You've studied the workings of the metabolism, looked at long-term approaches to improving your health and losing weight, and learned how altering your lifestyle may impact your health from the inside out. Let's now review your metabolic mastery journey and discuss what lies ahead for a happier, healthier you.

Your Path to Metabolic Expertise

Your desire for change—to escape the cycle of restrictive diets, unsustainable weight reduction techniques, and dissatisfaction with your body's reaction to conventional treatments—was the starting point of your path toward metabolic mastery. By learning about metabolism and realizing that genuine mastery is found in balance and feeding rather than deprivation and restriction, you took the first step toward change.

In Chapter 1, you learn about the dangers of conventional diets, the yo-yo dieting cycle, and the unstated costs of metabolic damage. You realize that diets are ineffective over the long term and that concentrating solely on weight loss at the expense of metabolic health sets one up for long-term failure.

In Chapter 2, you learned about the metabolic solution, which emphasizes knowing macronutrients, eating for metabolic health, and acknowledging the role of hormones in metabolism. You acquired the knowledge and skills necessary to provide your body with the fuel it needs for optimum health and vigor by adopting a balanced diet and understanding how to assist your body's natural metabolic processes.

In Chapter 3, you learned about the fundamentals of metabolic mastery, how to put together a balanced plate, and how important meal scheduling is. You realized that achieving metabolic mastery is about giving your body the nutrition it needs to flourish rather than about restriction or deprivation, and you discovered how to design a long-lasting eating schedule that complements your metabolic objectives.

In Chapter 4, you learned about foods that can speed up your metabolism, including superfoods, recipes to speed up your metabolism, and supplements to maintain your metabolism's health. To maximize your metabolic function, you discovered how to include nutrient-dense foods in your diet, try out new recipes, and make informed supplement decisions.

In Chapter 5, you looked at lifestyle choices for healthy metabolism, including the value of exercise, stress reduction methods, and getting enough sleep. You discovered how important it is to emphasize physical exercise, stress reduction, and enough sleep in your everyday life because these behaviors are critical to metabolic health.

In Chapter 6, you faced obstacles head-on, overcoming weight reduction plateaus, addressing metabolic resistance, and preserving metabolic health indefinitely. On the path to metabolic mastery, you discovered how to overcome setbacks, maintain motivation, and recognize your accomplishments.

Further Actions for a Happier, Healthier You

Having reached the pinnacle of metabolic mastery, it's now time to focus on the future and picture the happiest, healthiest version of yourself. Here are some things you should think about doing as you proceed on your journey to wellness:

1. **Remain Devoted to Your Routines**: Keep in mind that achieving metabolic mastery is a lifetime process

rather than a goal. Maintain your commitment to the long-term routines you've created, and keep putting your health and well-being first in all you do.

2. **Listen to Your Body**: Observe how your body reacts to various diets, workout regimens, and way of life decisions. Make decisions that support your specific metabolic demands, pay attention to your body's signals of hunger and fullness, and respect your body's need for rest and recuperation.

3. **Continue Learning and Developing**: The study of nutrition and metabolism is a dynamic field, so maintain an open mind and a curious attitude. Continue researching new studies, trying out different diets and workout regimens, and looking for chances to advance your development.

4. **Give Your Knowledge and Experience**: Help others by sharing what you know and have experienced. Find methods to improve the lives of others, whether it is by volunteering in your community, encouraging healthy living practices, or helping a friend on their wellness path.

5. **Celebrate Your Progress**: Lastly, give yourself a moment to reflect on your accomplishments and how far you've come. No matter how little your victory was,

remember to celebrate it and the effort and commitment it took to get there. You'll be inspired and encouraged to keep aiming for your best self if you celebrate your accomplishments and pay tribute to your path.

As you turn the last page of "Metabolic Mastery: Ditch Your Diet, Shed Fat, and Maintain a Healthy Lifestyle," remember that you are equipped with the information, resources, and frame of mind you need to succeed on your metabolic mastery path. Accept the strength of long-lasting routines, maintain your fortitude in the face of difficulties, and never give up on becoming a better, happier version of yourself. Your metabolic mastery journey is just getting started, and there are countless opportunities for change.